MommyHooray Presents:

The Expectations

The Quiet Pressure Beneath the Surface

by MommyHooray

MommyHooray Presents: The Expectations
by MommyHooray

Written and published under the pen name MommyHooray.
Illustrations created using digital illustration tools.

Printed in the United States of America.

ISBN: 978-1-972071-43-4

For more stories and updates, visit:
https://sites.google.com/view/mommyhooray

This is for the part of you
that keeps going
even when it's tired.

The part that shows up,
again and again.

That part is strong.
That part is enough.

And that part of you
is allowed to rest,
without losing your worth.

With Googolplex Love,

MommyHooray

You didn't choose all of this.

It built slowly—
in comments,
in silence,
in the things you felt you had to become.

Somewhere along the way,
"do your best" turned into "be everything."

Now you carry expectations you never agreed to...
but somehow still feel responsible for.

This is for that weight.
The one you feel— even when no one else sees it.

You wake up already behind.

Not because you are...
but because there's a version of you
you think you're supposed to be
waiting in the other room.

She's calmer.
More organized.
Less tired.

You chase her all day
and still feel like you missed her.

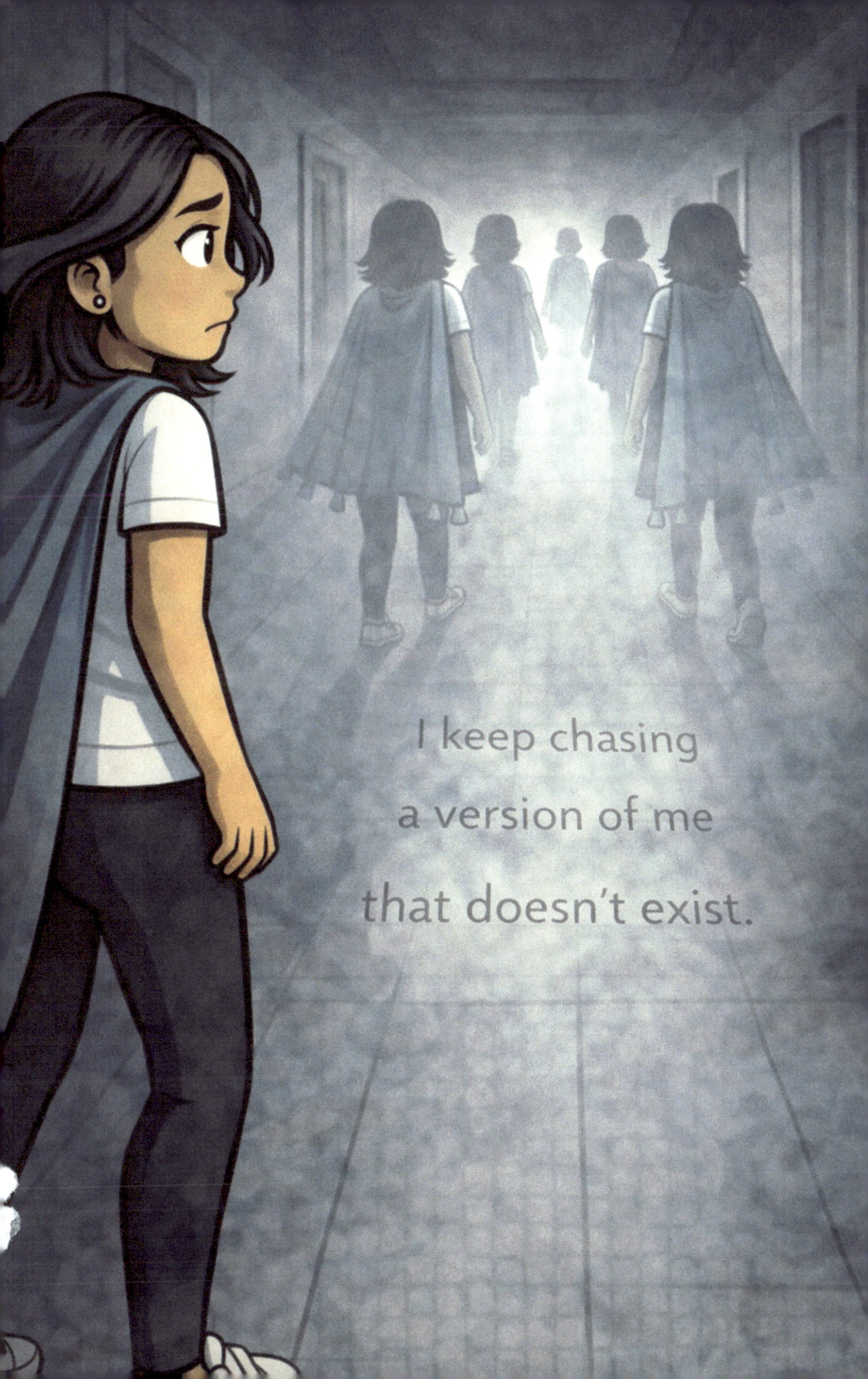
I keep chasing
a version of me
that doesn't exist.

You pack the snacks.
Remember the forms.
Answer the texts.

And still—
you feel like you forgot something.

Because no one told you the list never ends.

It just... grows quieter
and heavier.

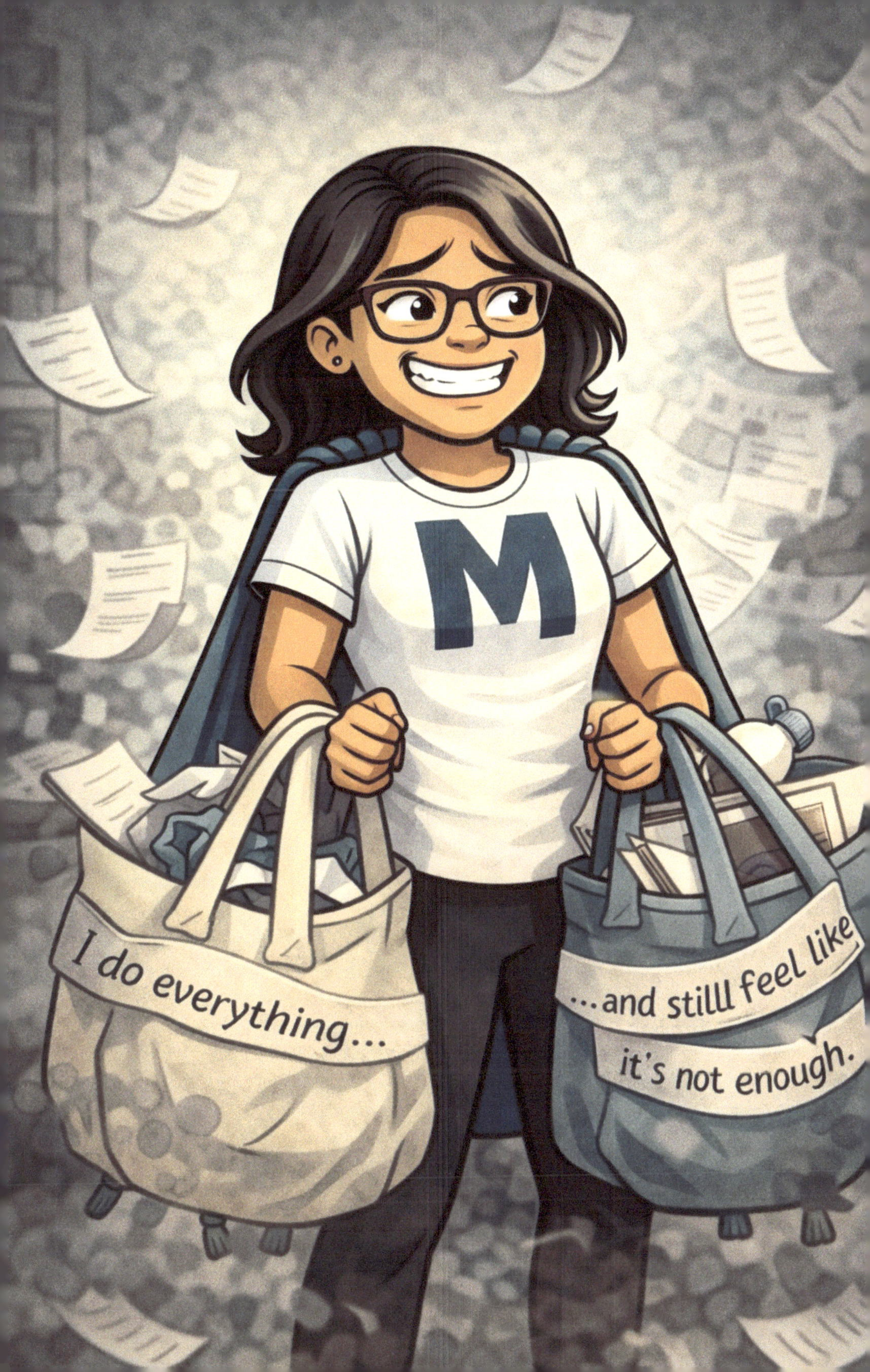
M
I do everything...
...and stilll feel like
it's not enough.

You say yes

before you even pause long enough

to check in with yourself.

Because saying no

feels like letting something fall—

even when the thing you're dropping is you.

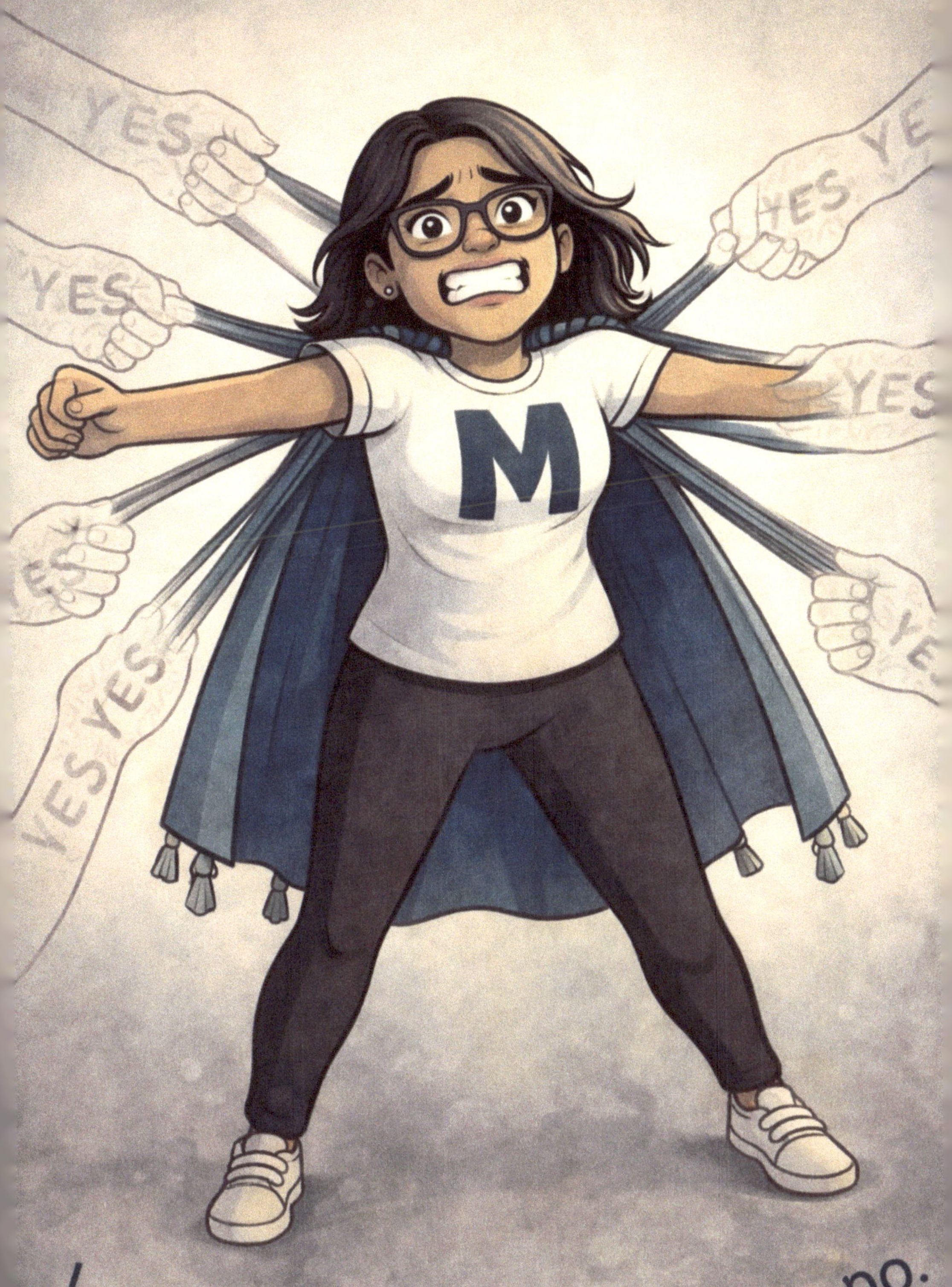

I say yes... even when I mean no.

You try to be patient.

Even when your body is loud,
and your mind is crowded,
and your energy is gone.

Because "good moms" don't snap.

So you swallow it—
until it spills anyway.

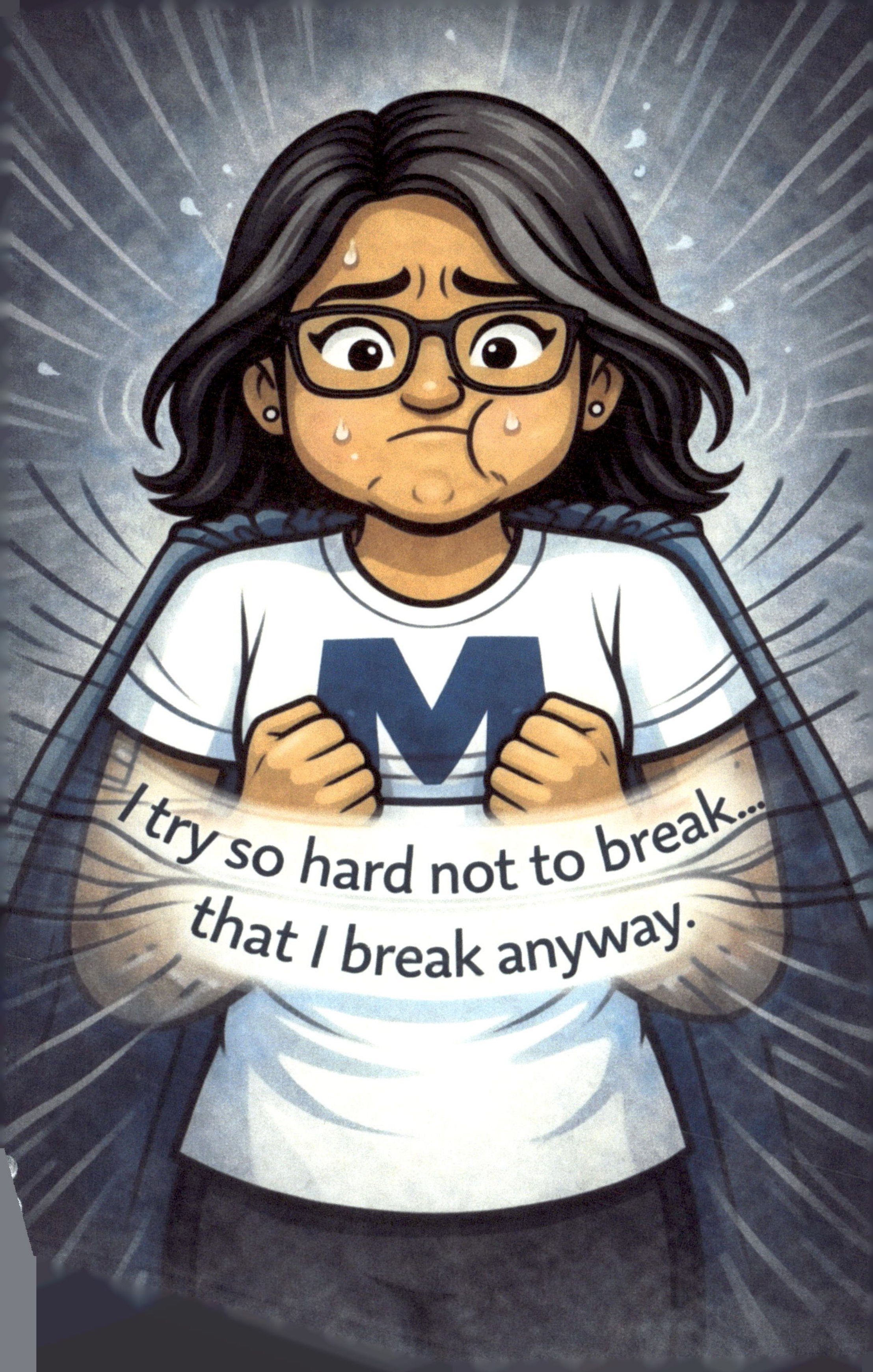
M
I try so hard not to break...
that I break anyway.

You make it look easy,
even when it isn't.

And because no one sees
the effort behind your normal,
they start to expect it—
every time.

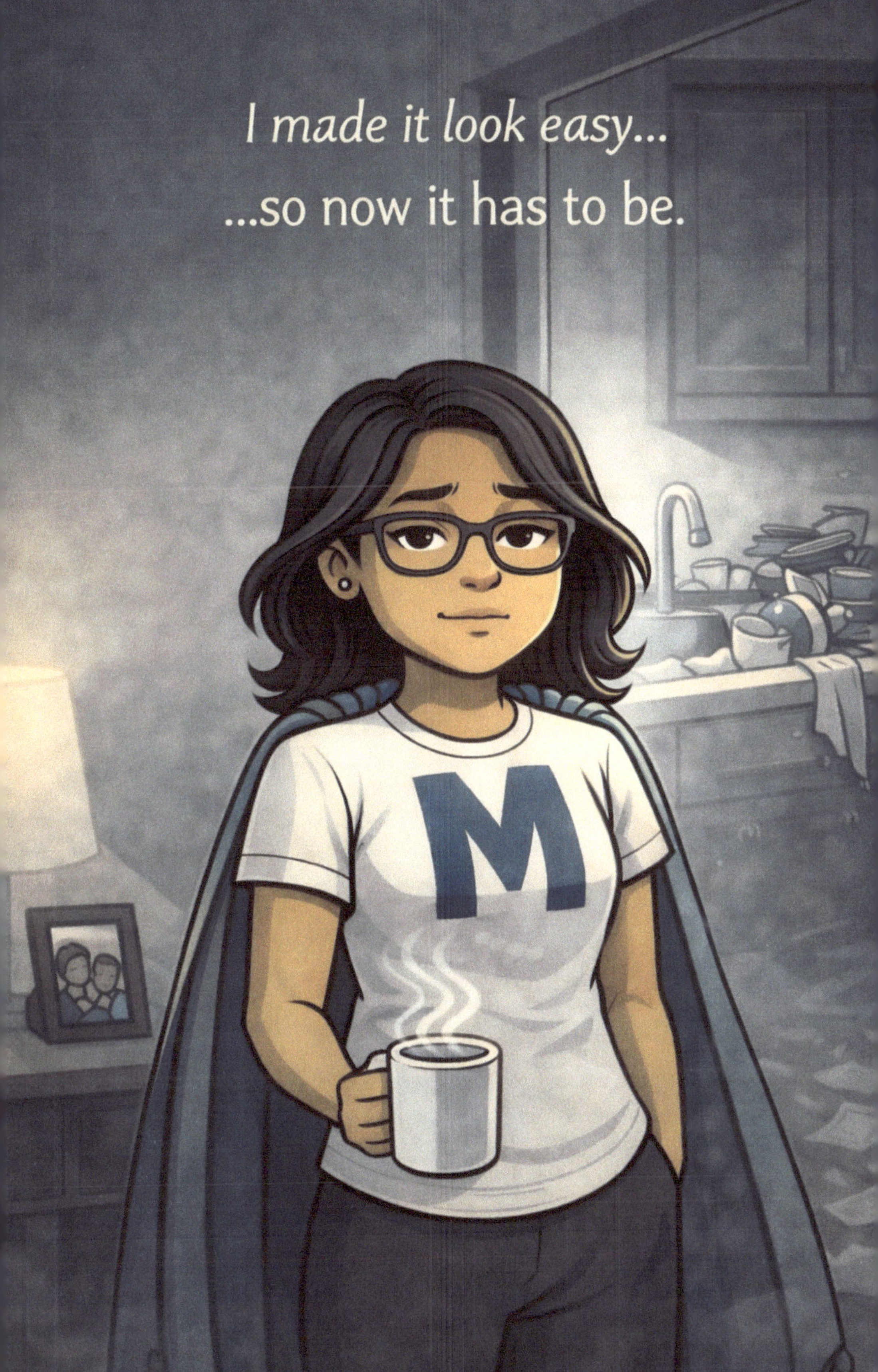
I made it look easy...
...so now it has to be.
M

You compare your everyday life
to a highlight reel
you never chose to watch.

And still—
you're the one who feels
like you're falling short.

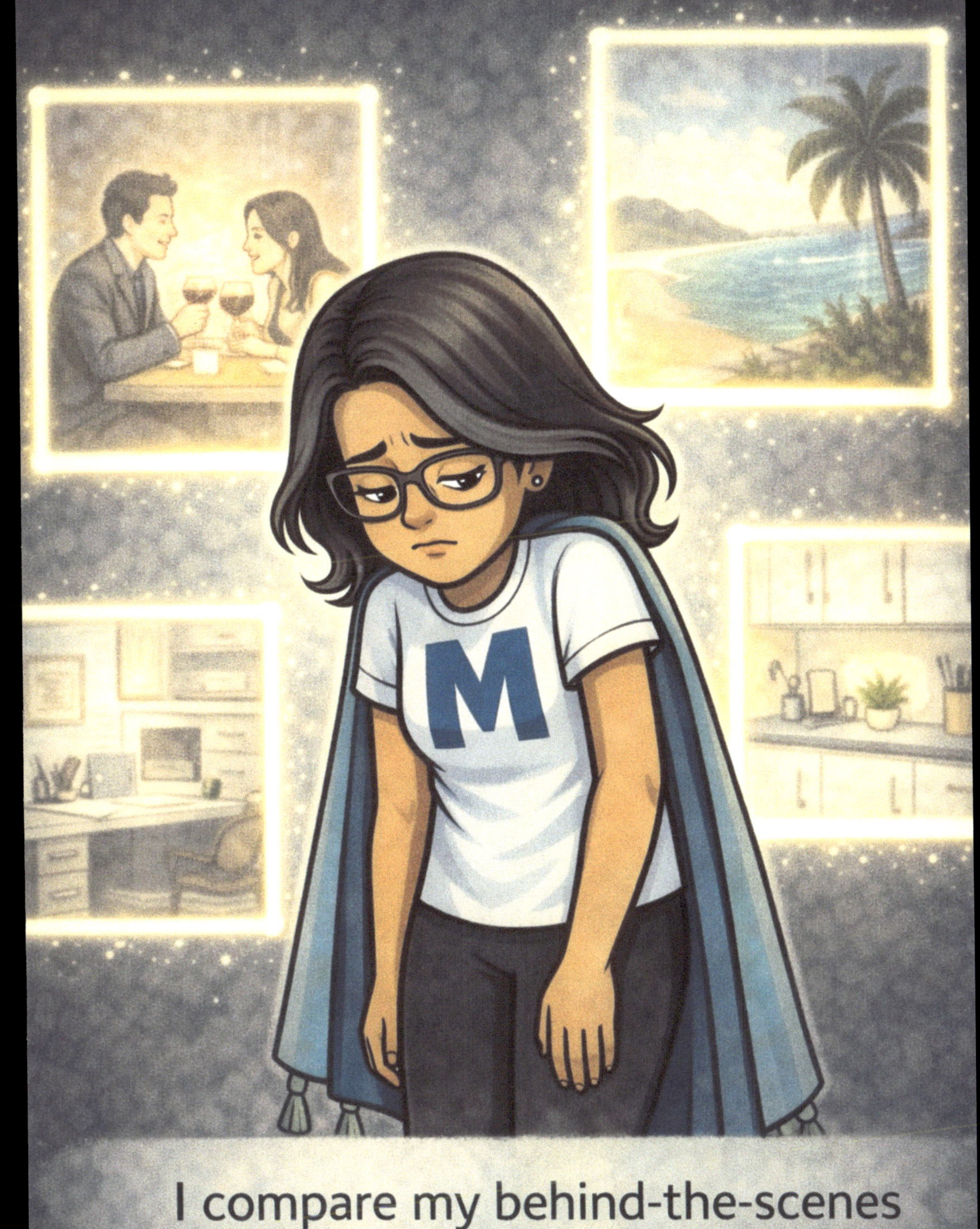
I compare my behind-the-scenes
to someone else's best moment.

You think rest has to be earned.

So even when you stop—
you don't really rest.

You just sit there,
feeling like you should be doing more.

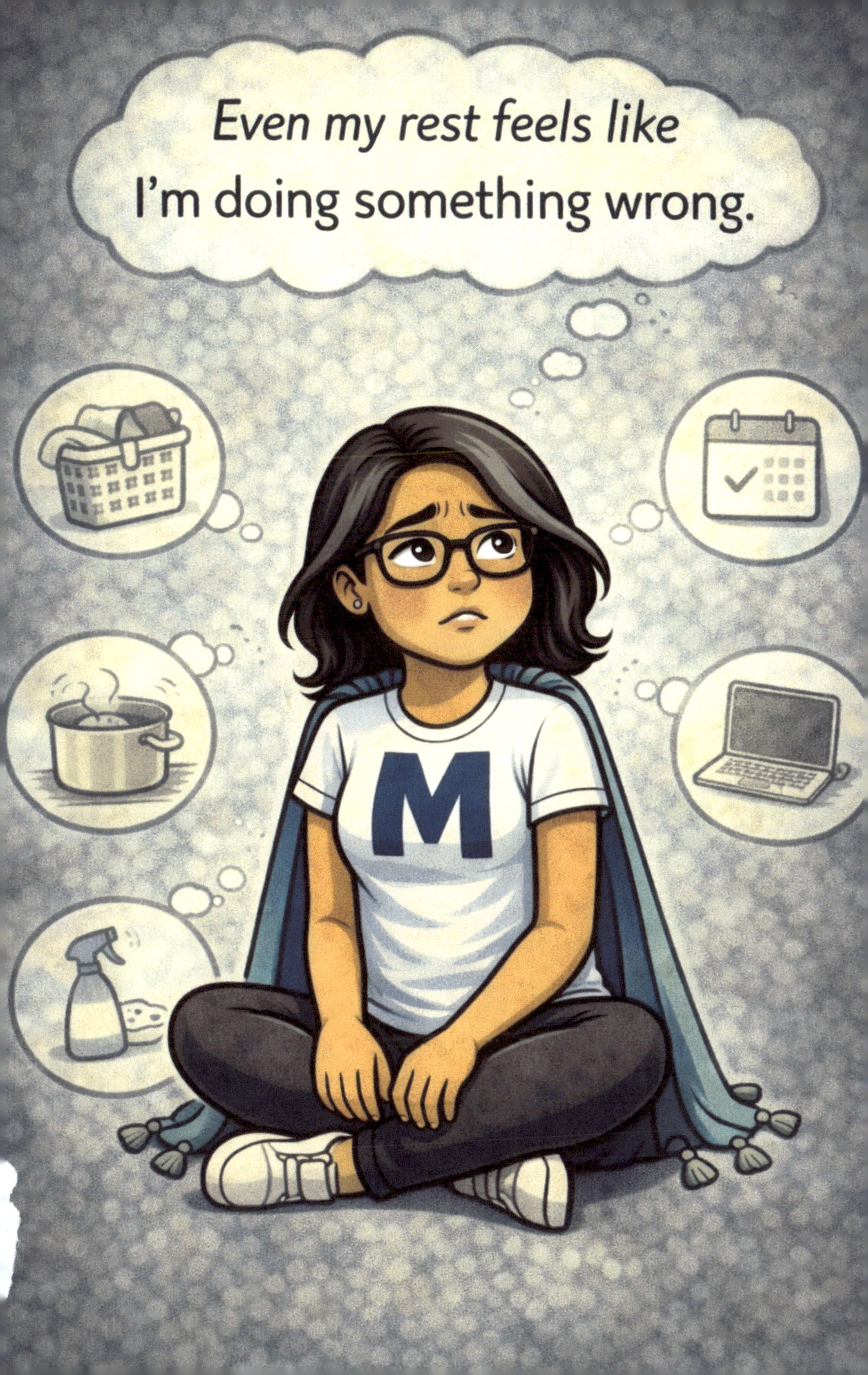

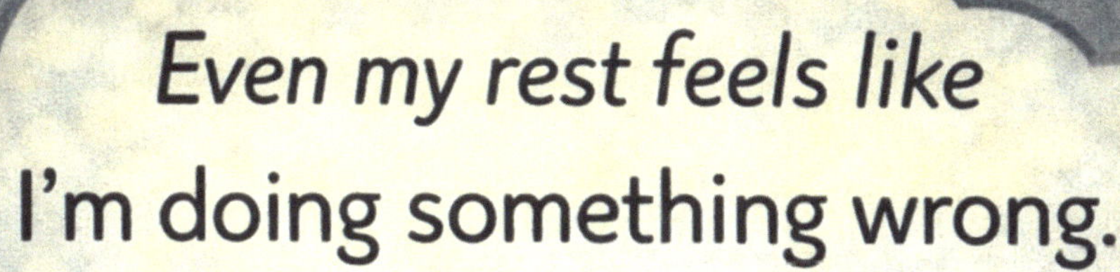
Even my rest feels like
I'm doing something wrong.

You try to be everything.

Patient.

Present.

Productive.

Put together.

All at once.

And when you can't—

you blame yourself.

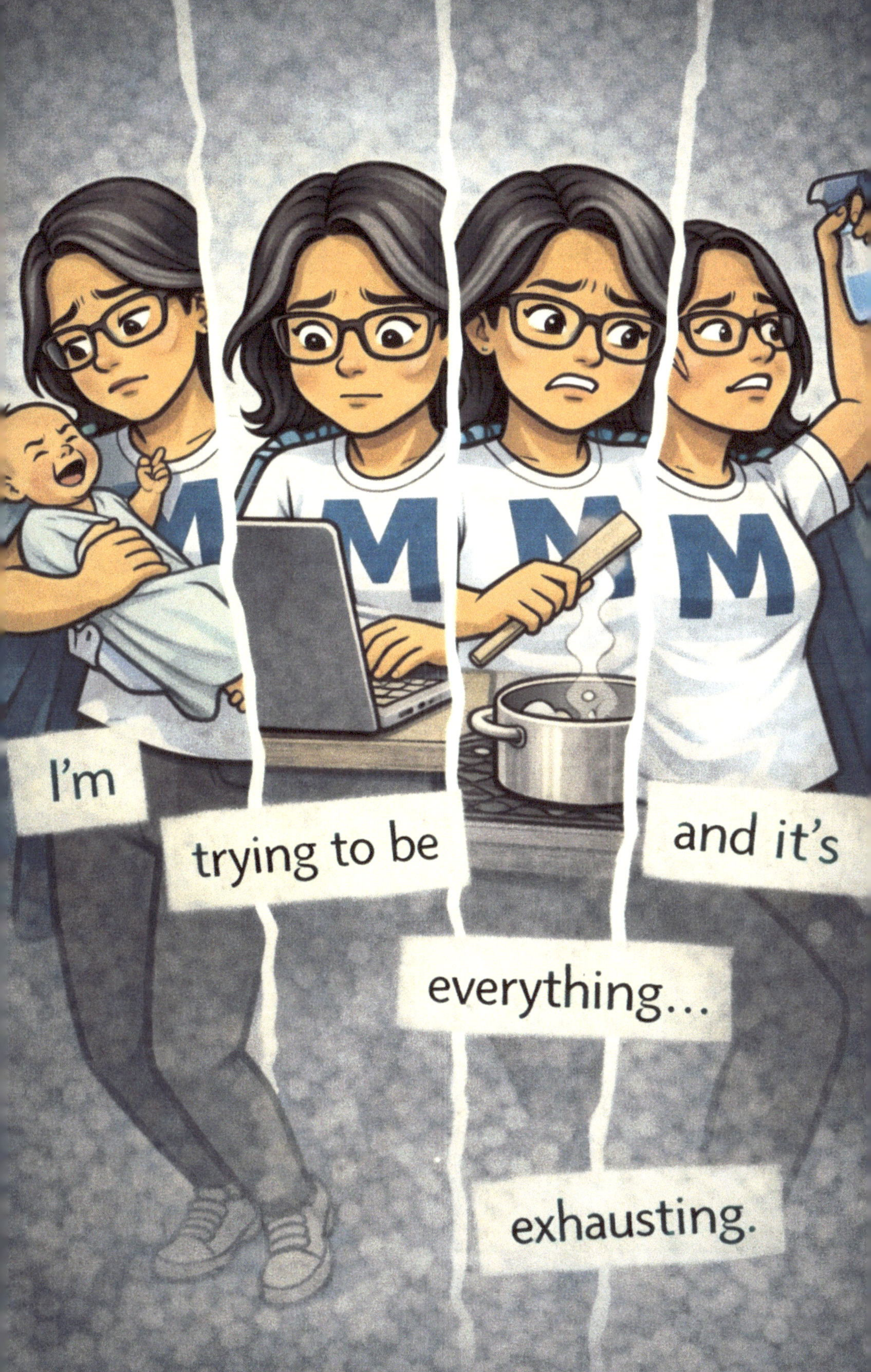
I'm
trying to be
and it's
everything...
exhausting.

You hear the voice:
“You should be better at this by now.”

It sounds convincing.

But it’s just pressure
that learned how to sound like you.

That voice in my head isn’t always mine.

You apologize

for things that don't need apologies.

Your tone.

Your timing.

Your limits.

As if existing needs permission.

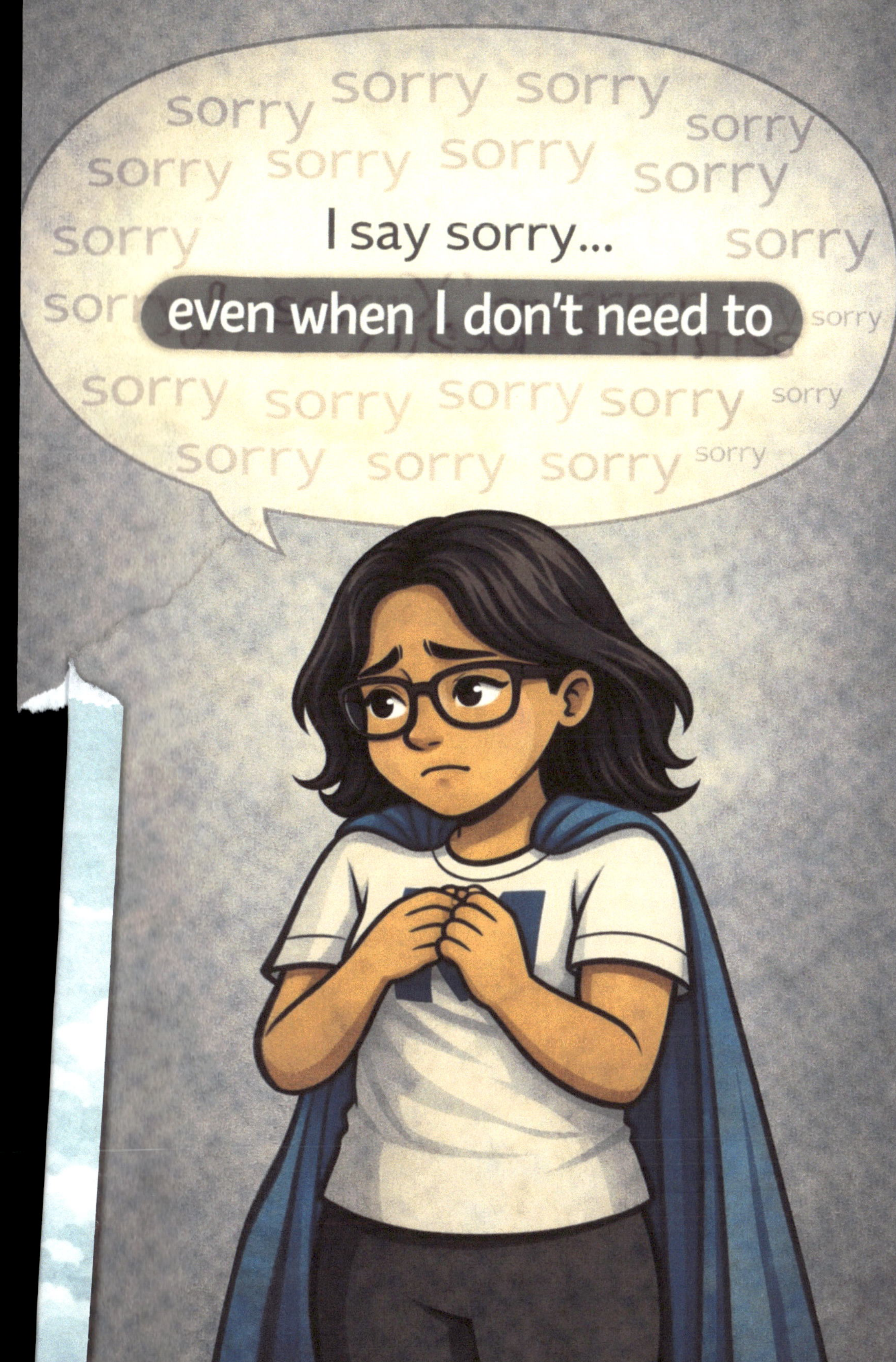

sorry sorry sorry
sorry
sorry sorry sorry sorry
sorry
I say sorry...
sorry
even when I don't need to
sorry
sorry sorry sorry sorry sorry
sorry sorry sorry sorry

You think if you just try harder—
you'll finally feel caught up.

But the finish line keeps moving.

So you keep going and still don't feel done.

No matter how much I do,
it never feels like enough.

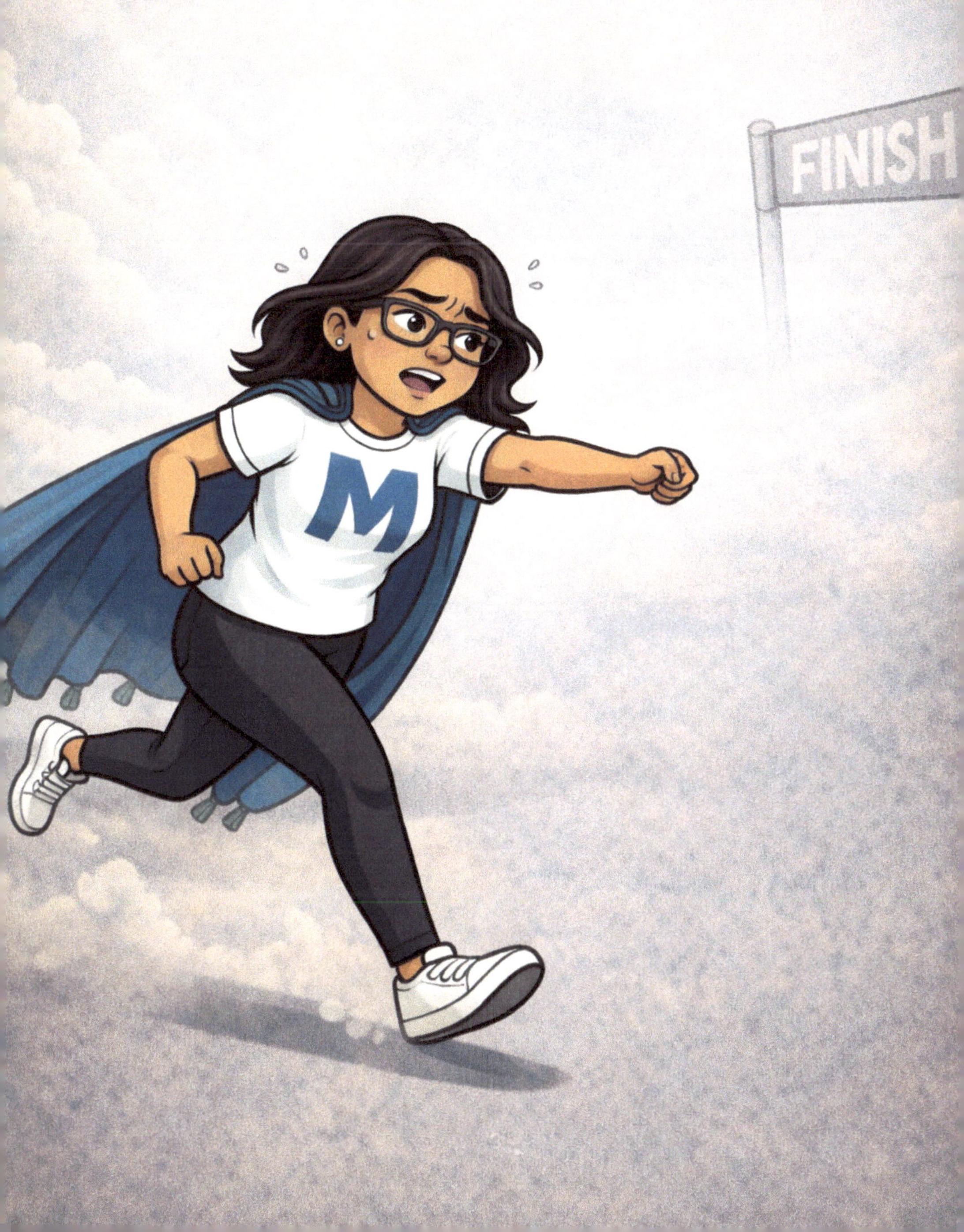

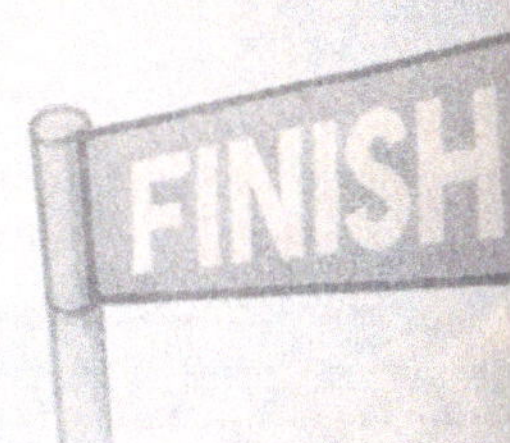

You hold yourself to a standard
you would never place on anyone else.

And call it discipline.

Even when it's heavy,
you tell yourself it's just what you should do.

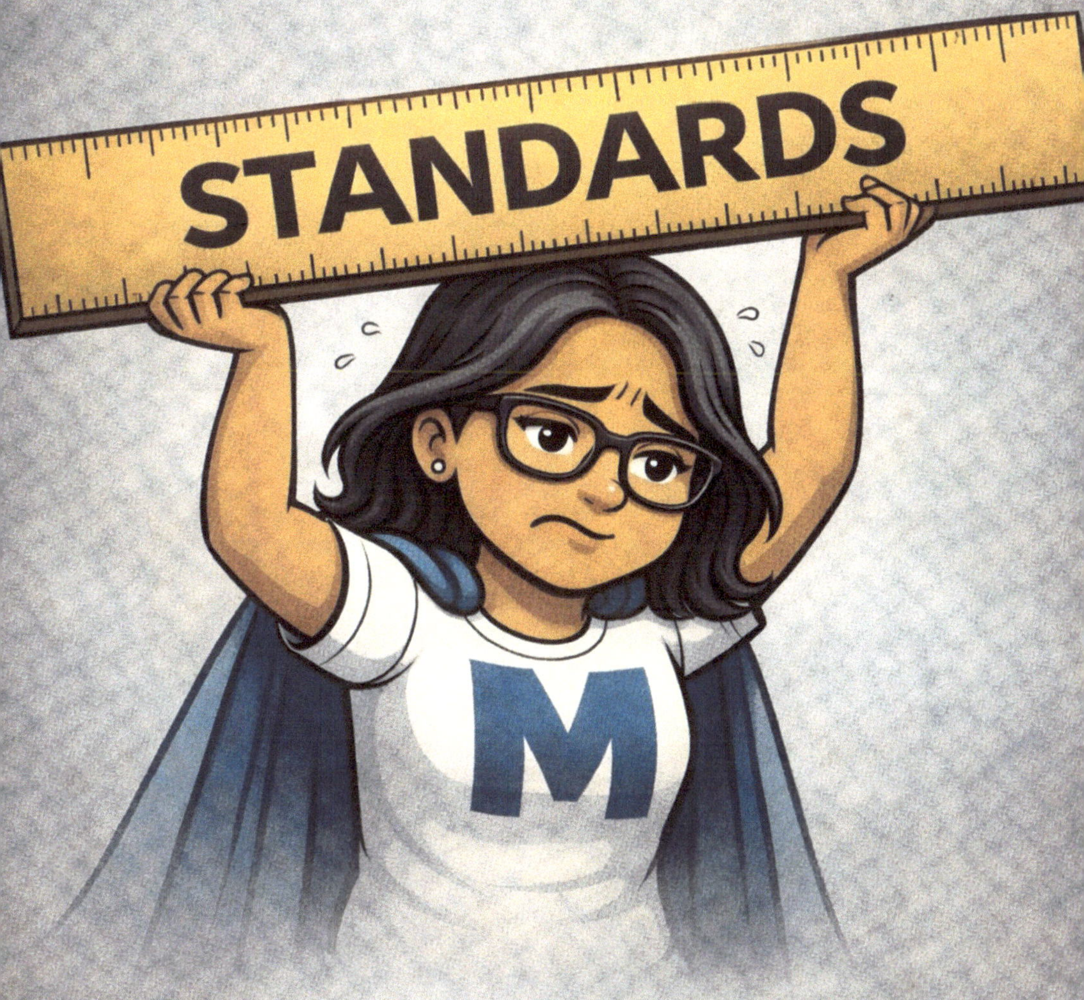

I'm harder on myself
than anyone else.

You feel guilty for needing help.
Even though you give it so freely.

You're the one people count on,
the one who figures it out.

So when you need something,
you downplay it—
like it shouldn't matter
as much as it does.

I give help easily...

but struggle to receive it.

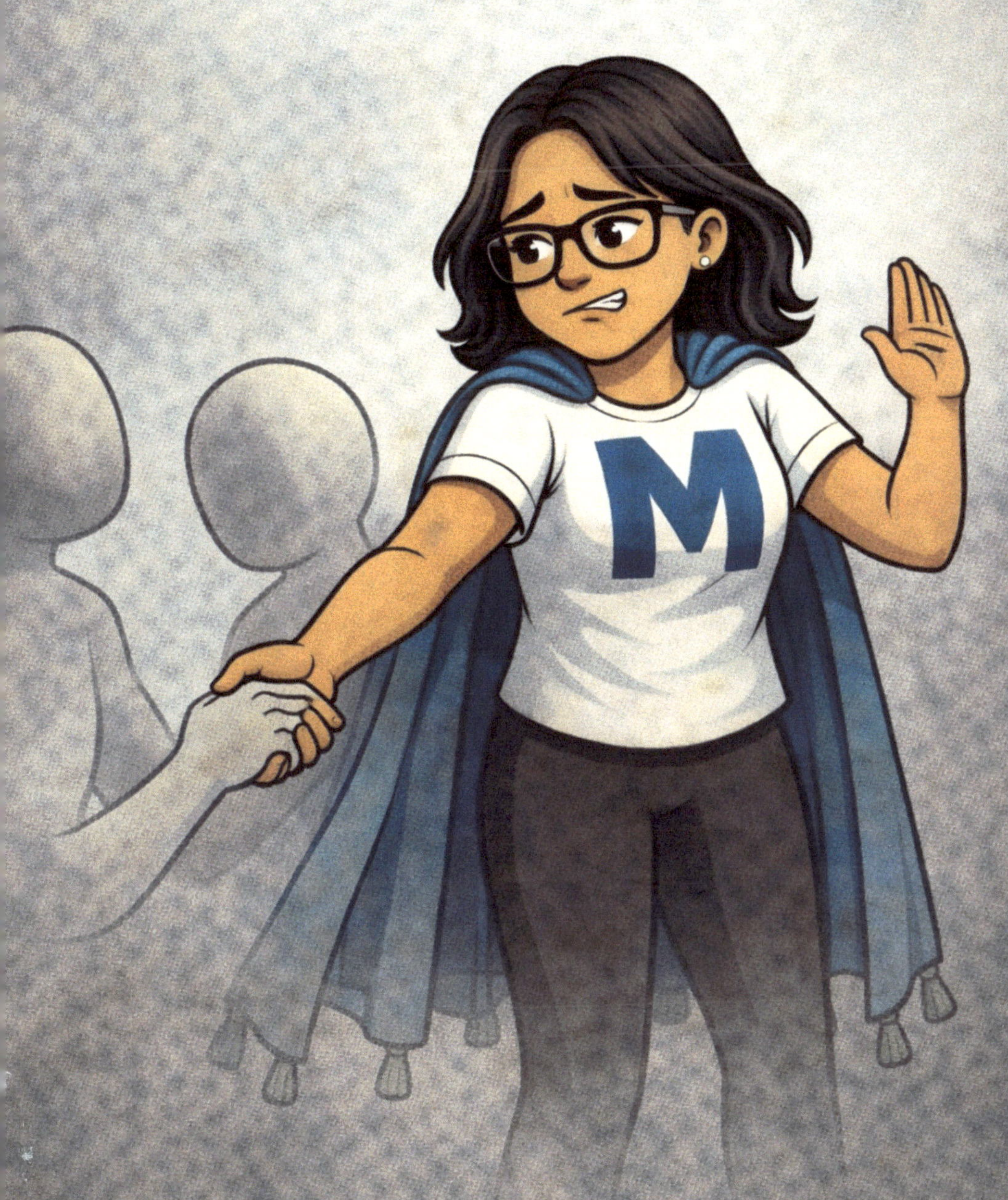

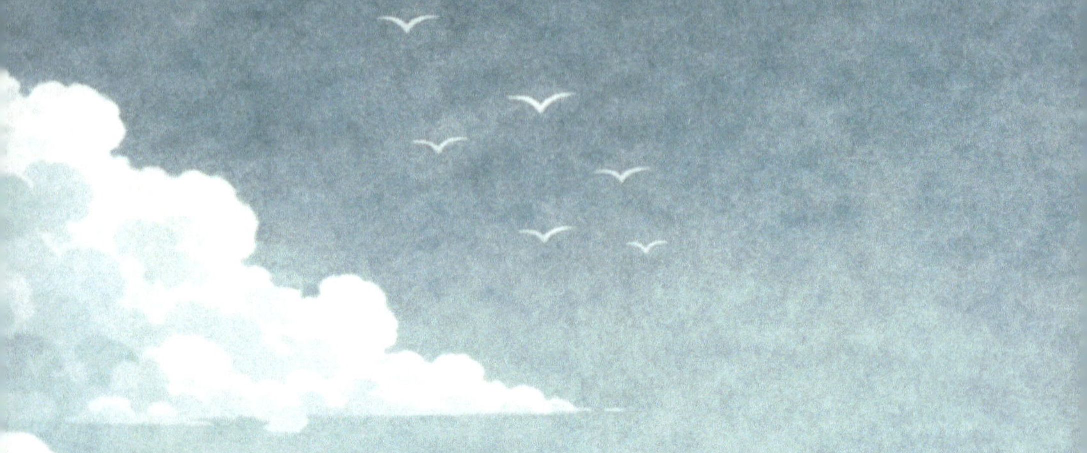

You think being overwhelmed
means you’re doing something wrong.

But maybe—
it means you’ve been carrying
more than you were meant to
on your own.

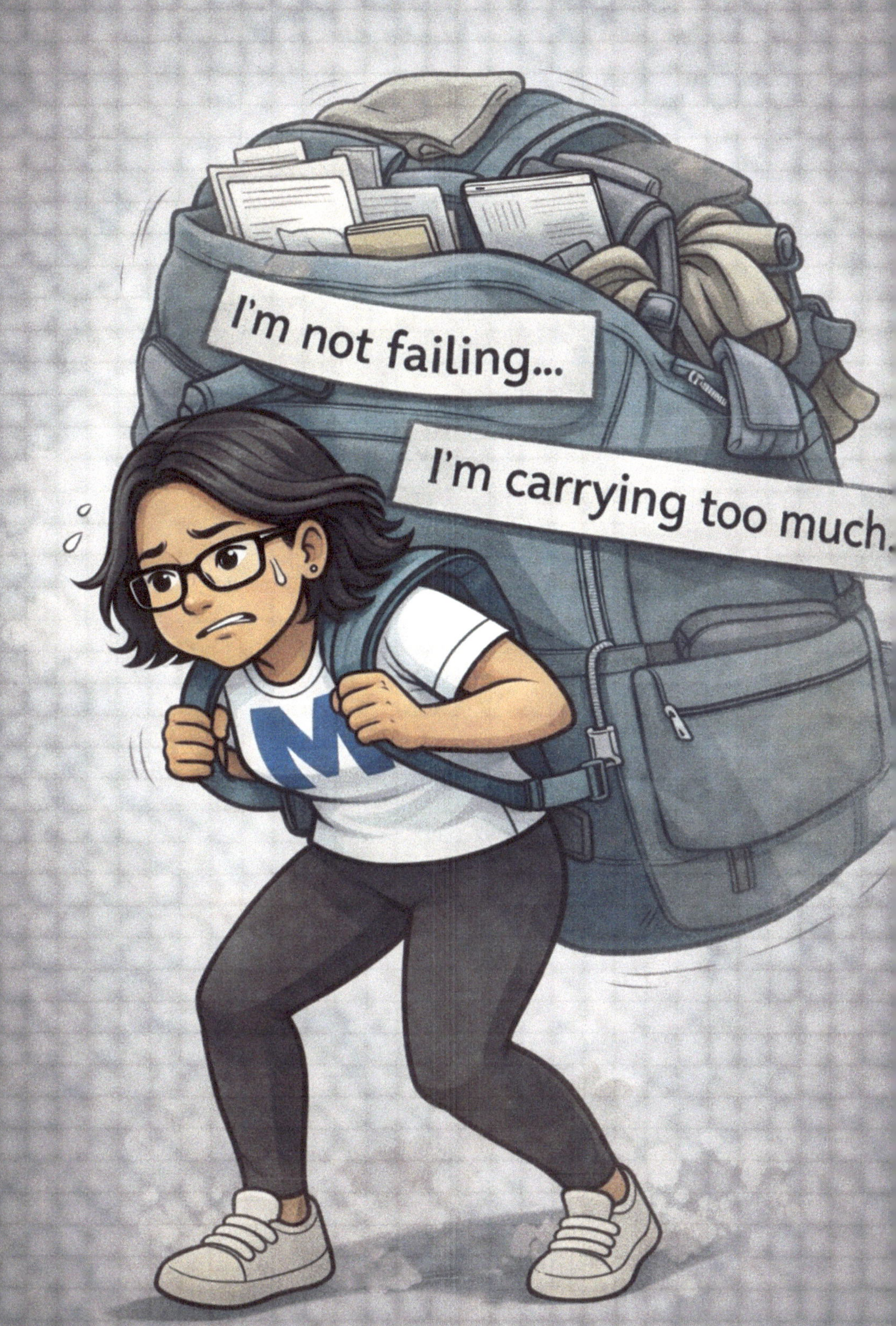
I'm not failing...
I'm carrying too much.

You try to control everything
so nothing falls apart.

So you carry more,
tighten your grip,
push a little harder.

But something still does—
you.

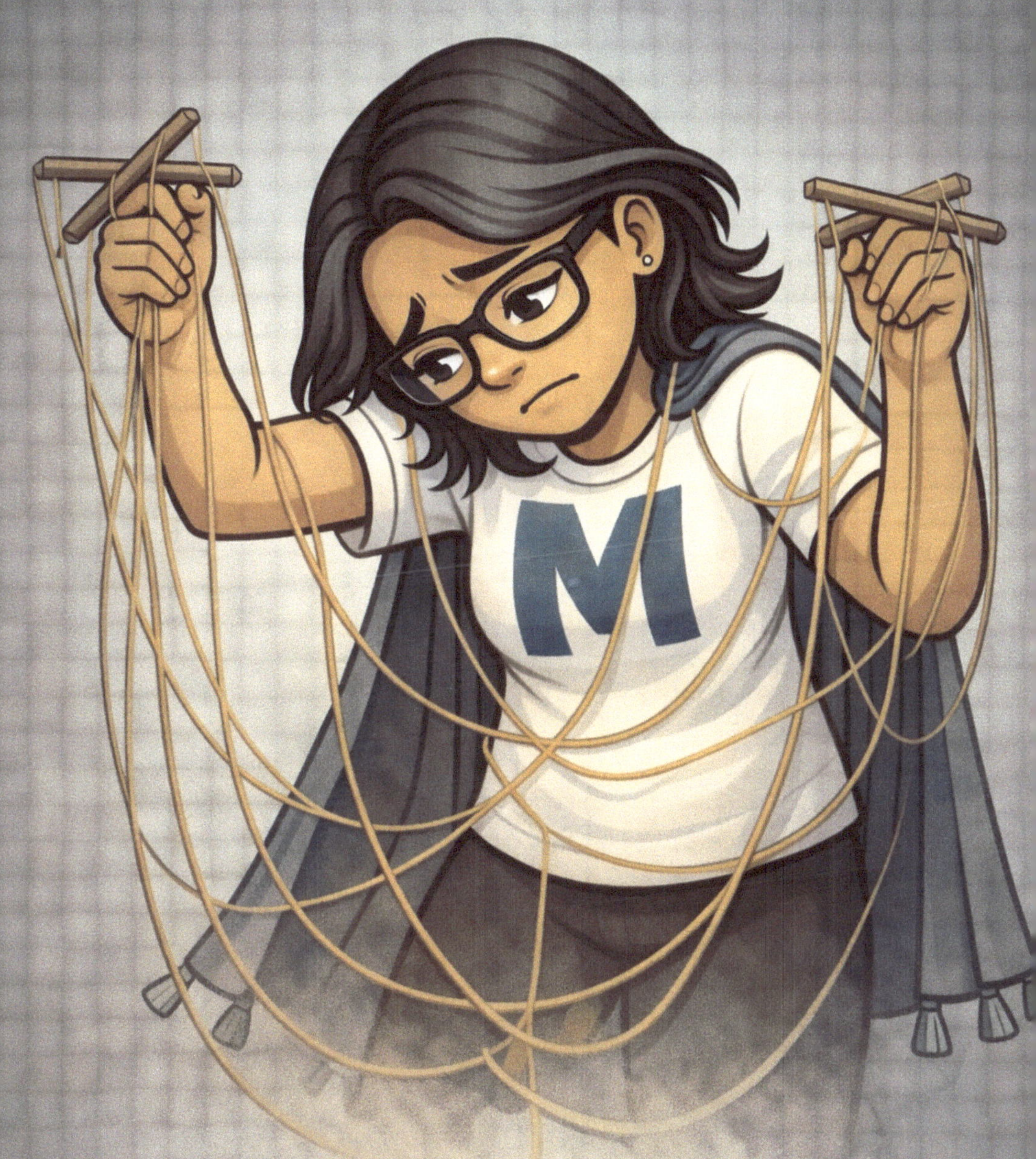

I try to hold everything together...

...and lose myself.

You measure your day by what didn't get done.
And forget everything that did.

As if the effort
somehow doesn't matter.

As if showing up
still isn't enough.

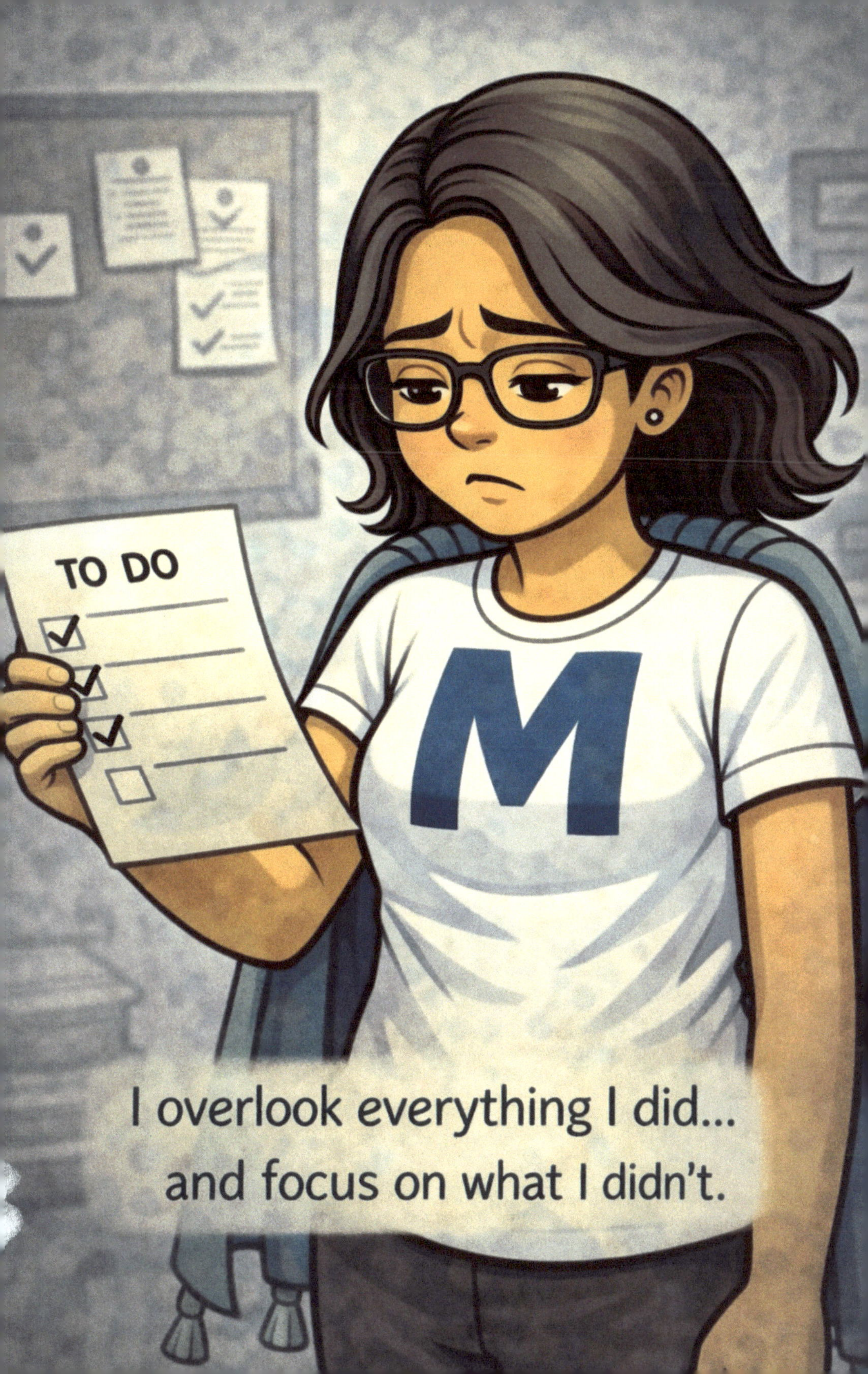
TO DO
M
I overlook everything I did...
and focus on what I didn't.

You think you're the only one
struggling like this.

Because everyone else
looks like they've figured it out.

But they haven't.

They're figuring it out too—
just not always out loud.

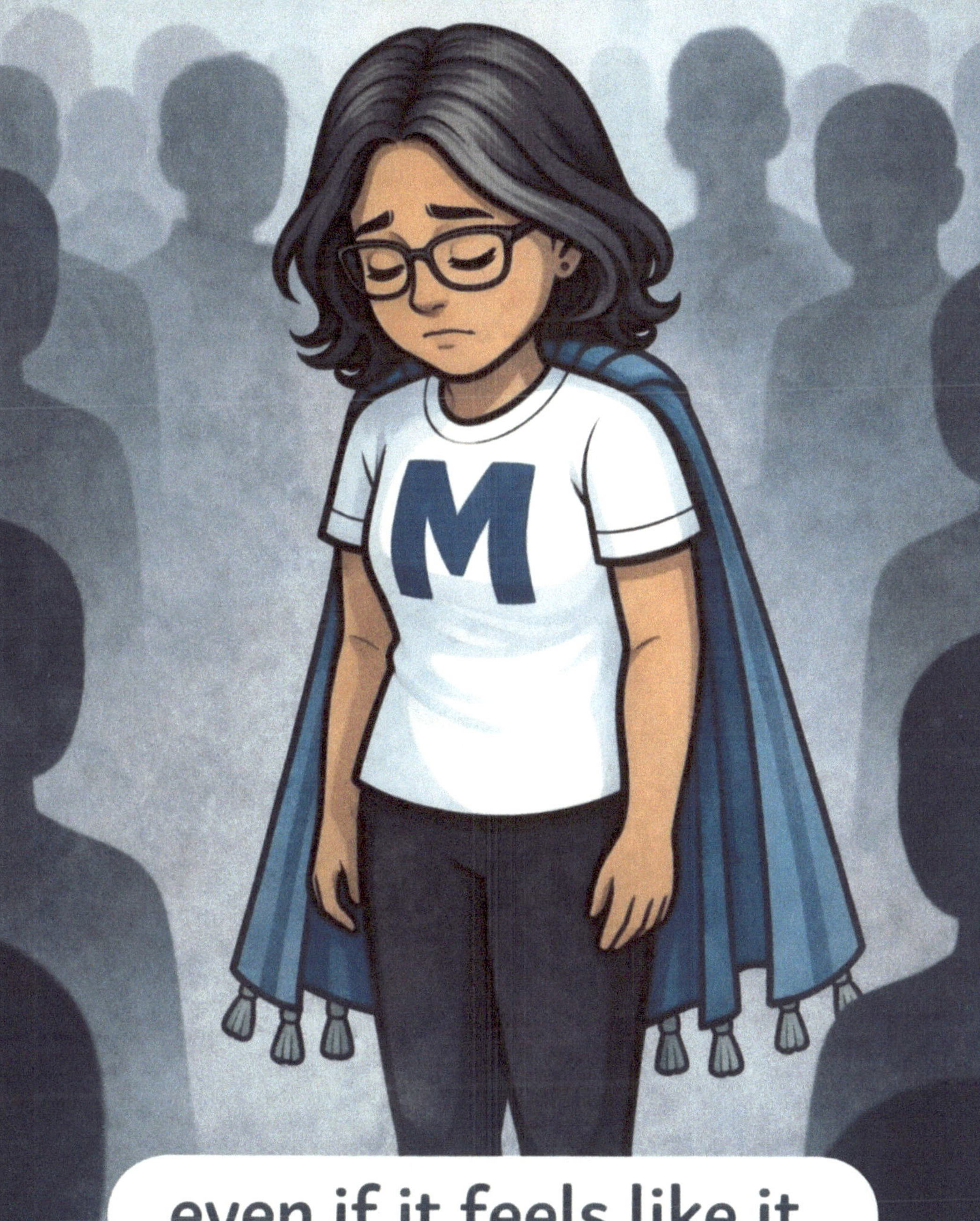
I'm not the only one...
even if it feels like it.
M

You keep raising the bar once you reach it.

So you never actually arrive.

Just one more thing,
one more step,
one more version of better.

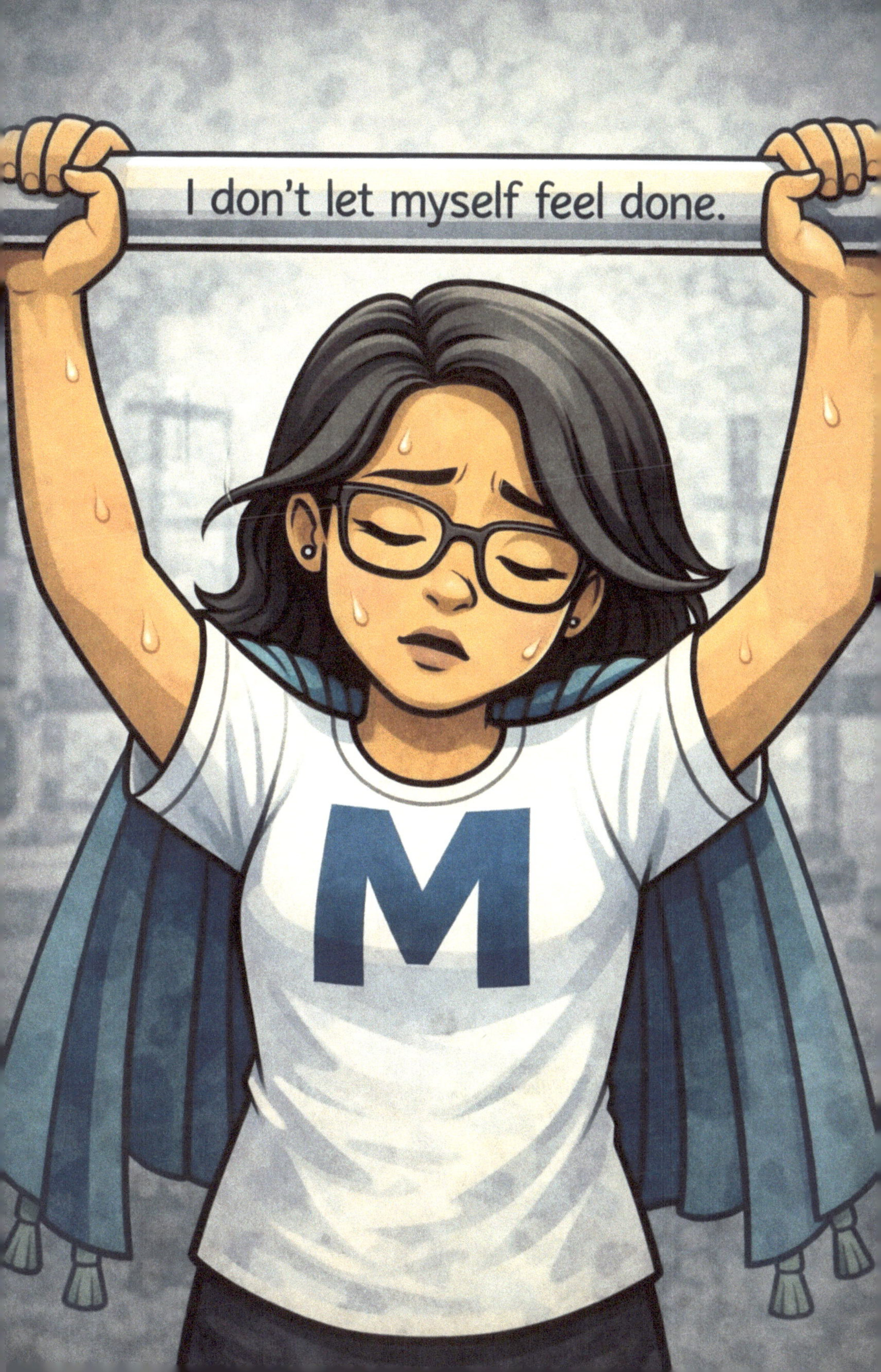
I don't let myself feel done.
M

You think slowing down
means falling behind.

But maybe—
it's the only way
to catch up with yourself.

To breathe again.
To feel a little more like you.

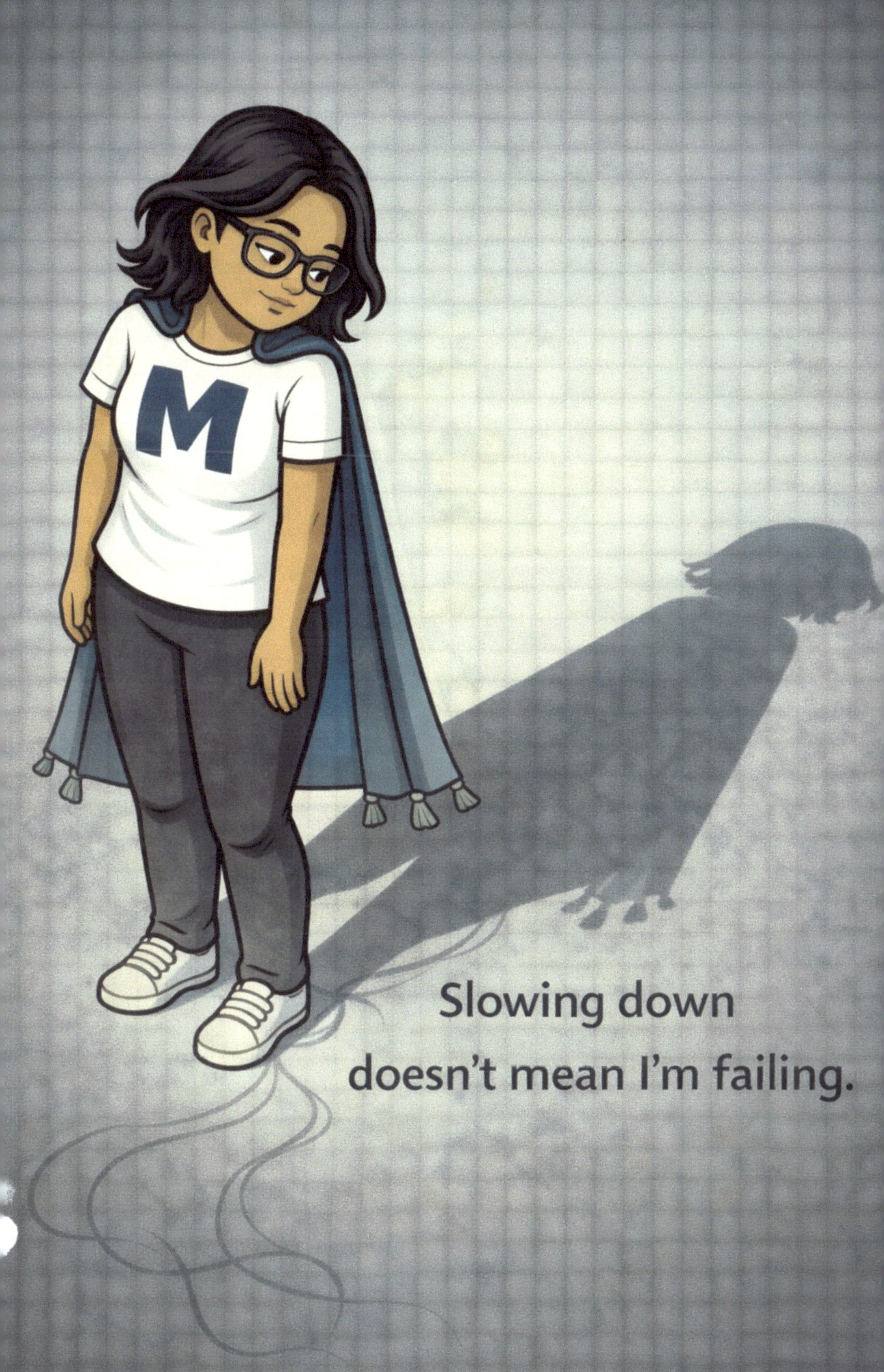
Slowing down
doesn't mean I'm failing.

You carry expectations
you never agreed to.

And call them responsibilities.

Like they just became yours
somewhere along the way.

Without you even noticing.

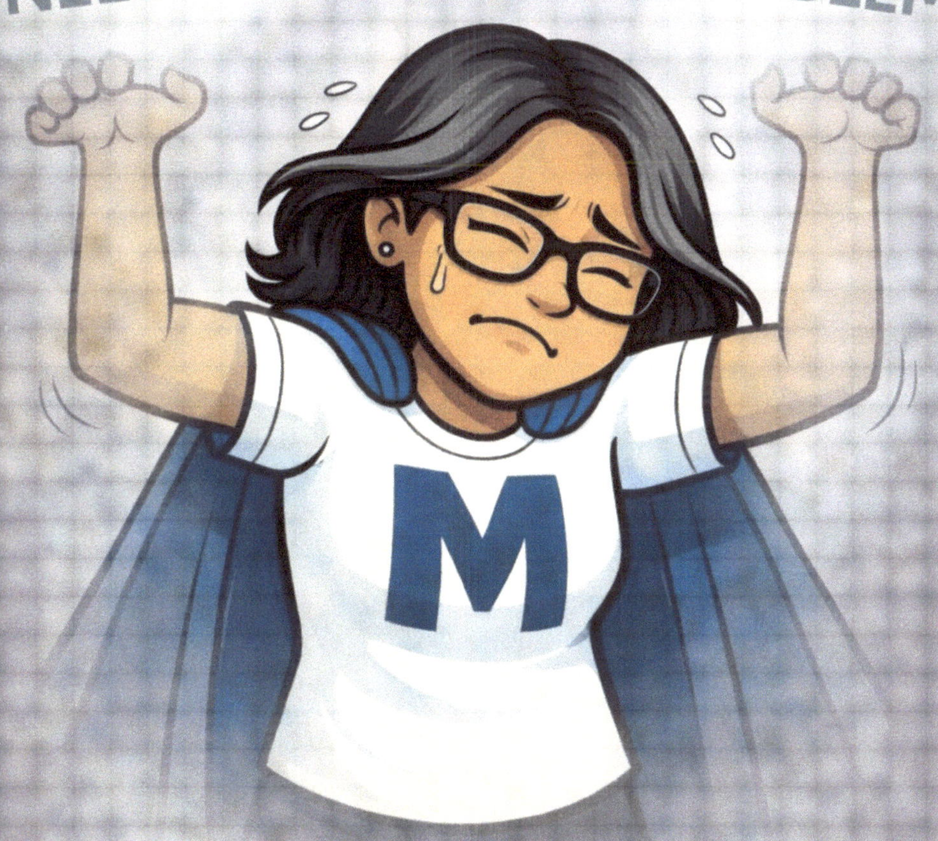

Not everything I carry
is mine to hold.

You think you have to prove
you're doing a good job.

But the people who matter most—
already feel it.

They don't need perfection.
They just need you.

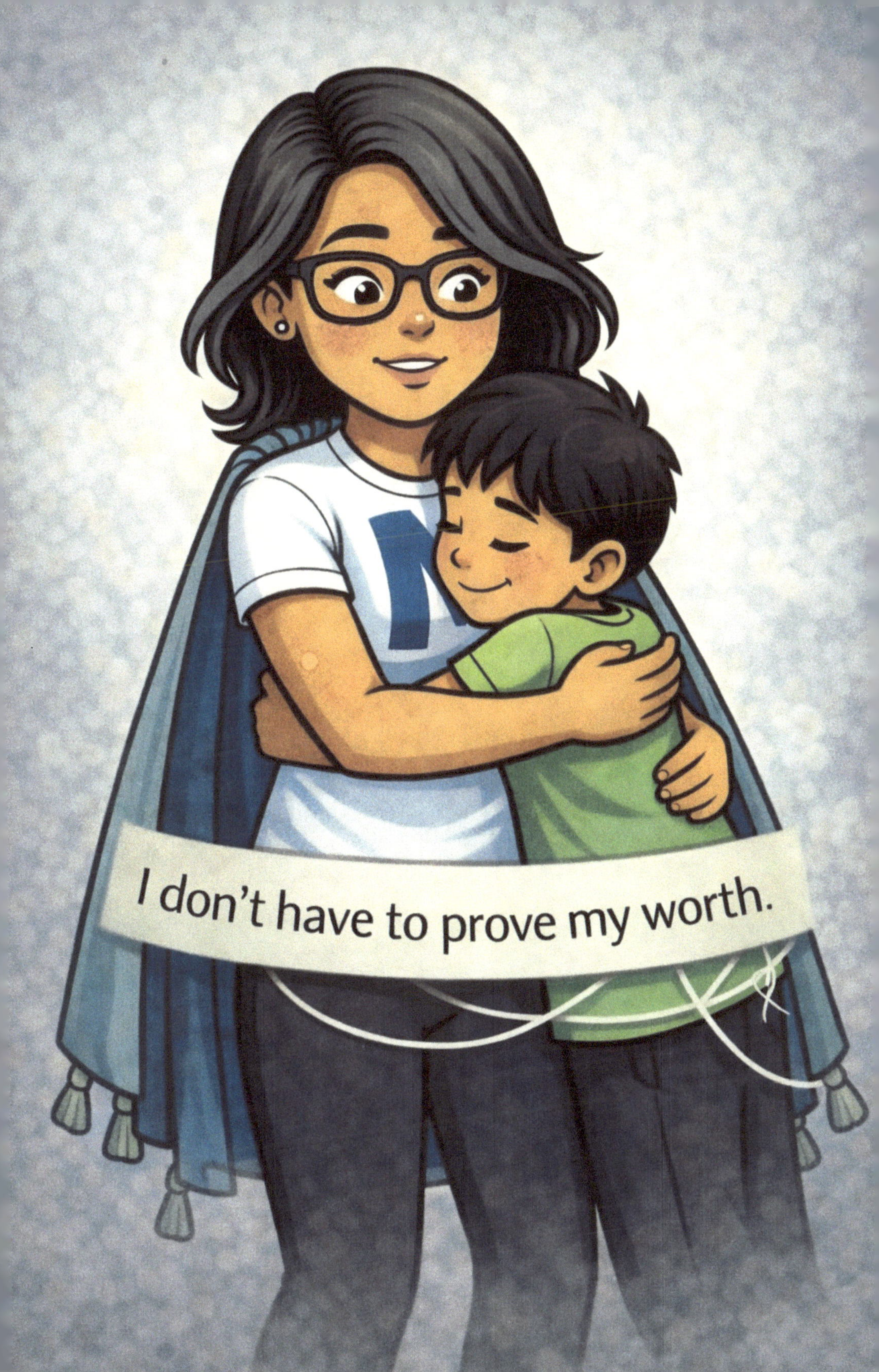
I don't have to prove my worth.

You are not behind.
You are not failing.
You are not less.

You are just carrying a story
that was never meant to be this heavy.

And you can set it down.

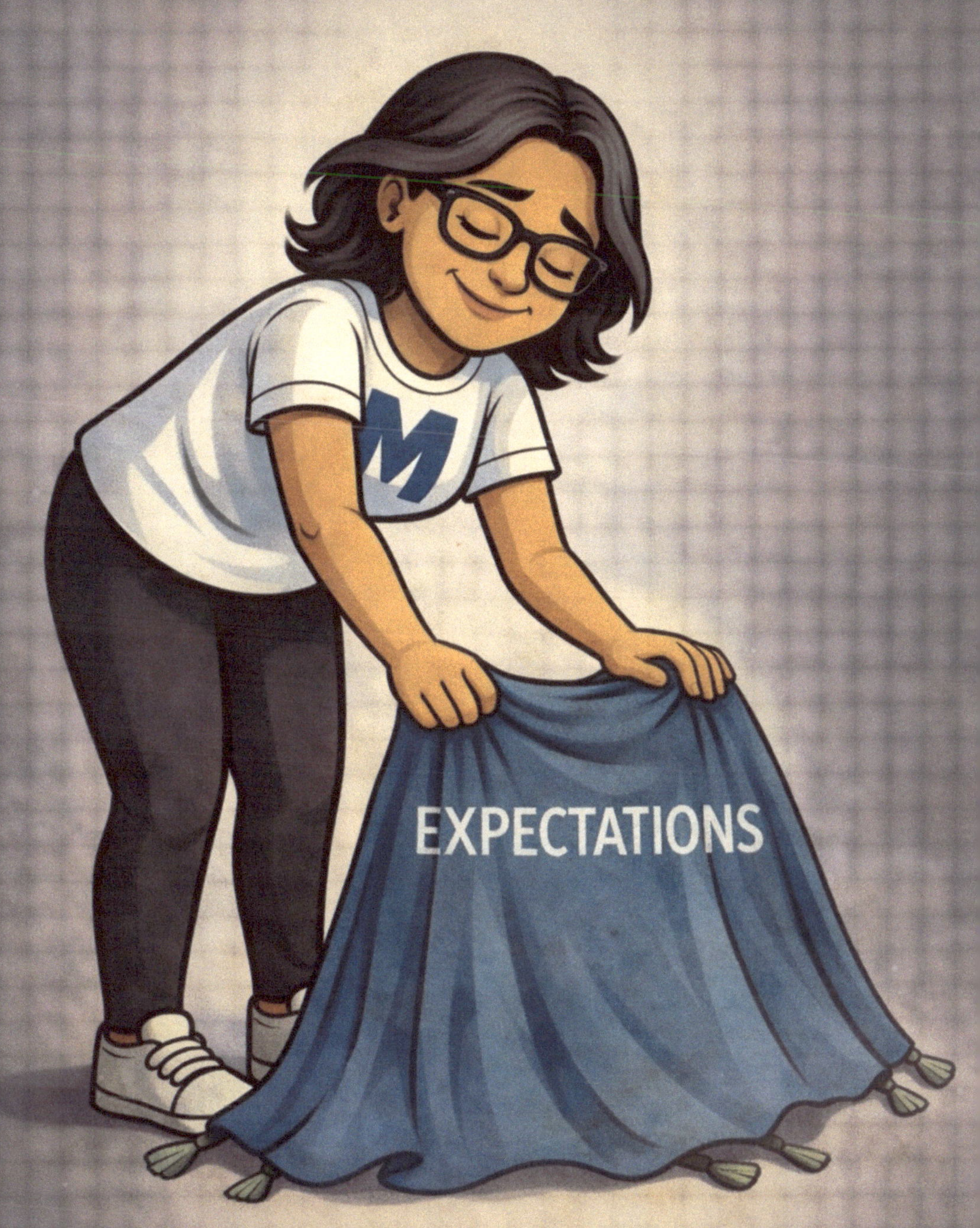
EXPECTATIONS
I'm allowed to put this down.

Not everything you carry belongs to you.

Some of it is noise.
Some of it is habit.
Some of it... you can let go.

You don't have to prove you're enough.
You don't have to earn your rest.

You already are.

And whatever you choose to keep—
let it leave room for you, too.♡

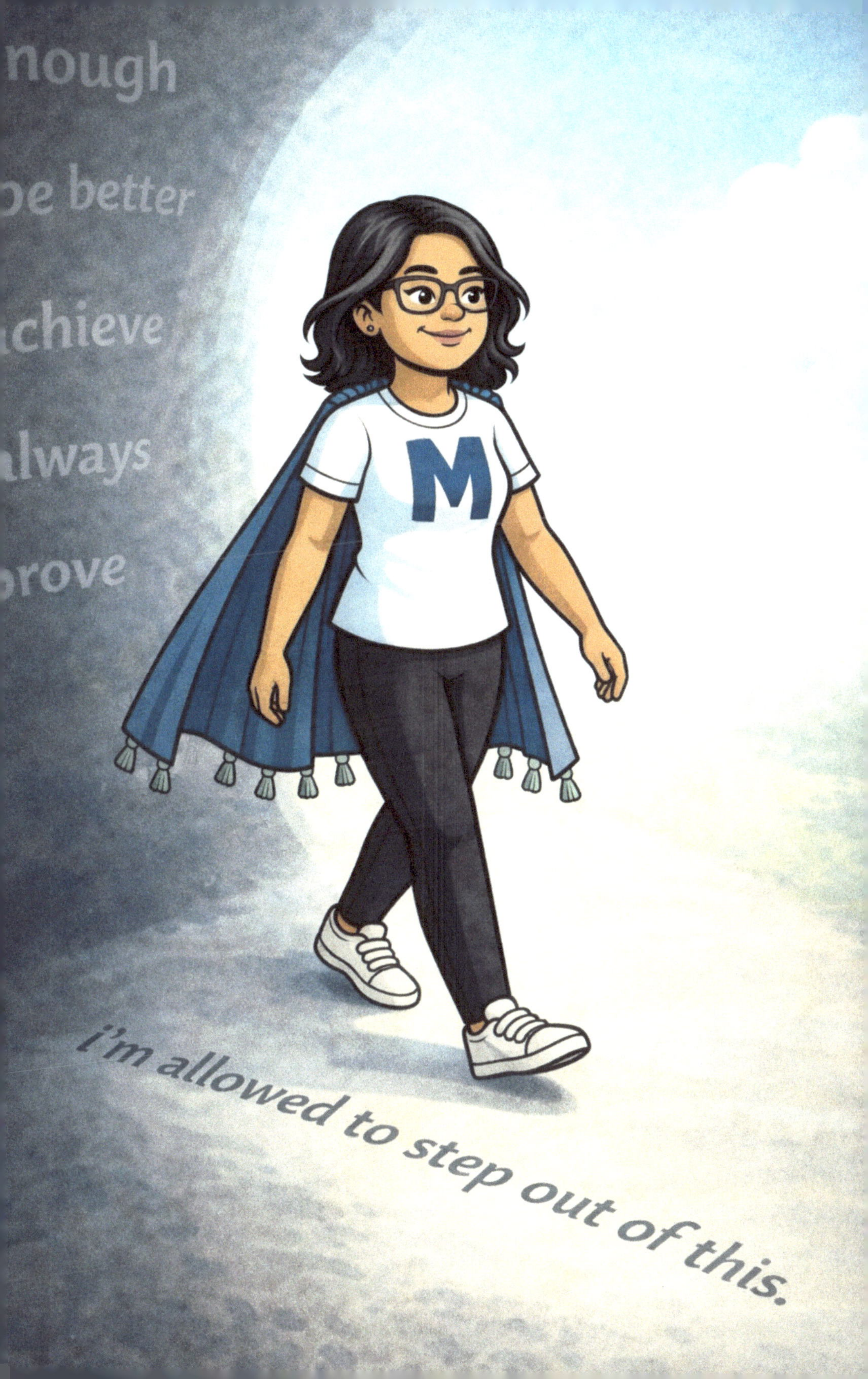

nough

e better

chieve

lways

rove

i'm allowed to step out of this.

Also by MommyHooray

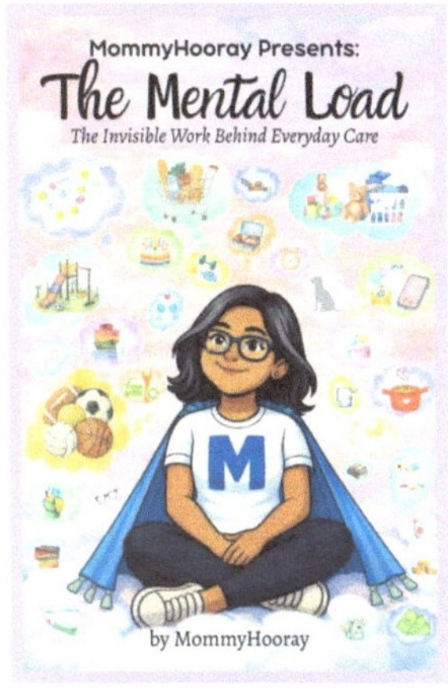

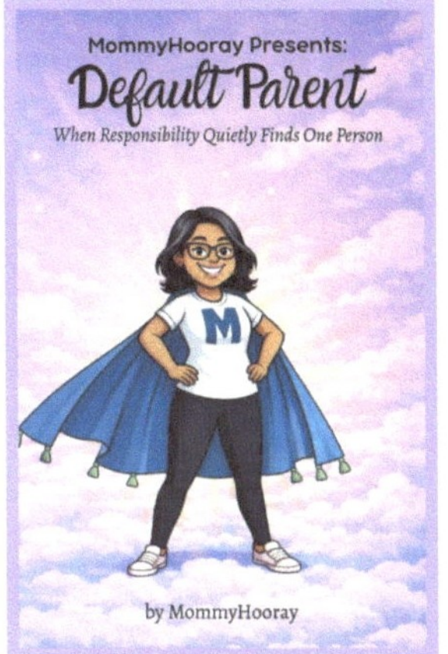

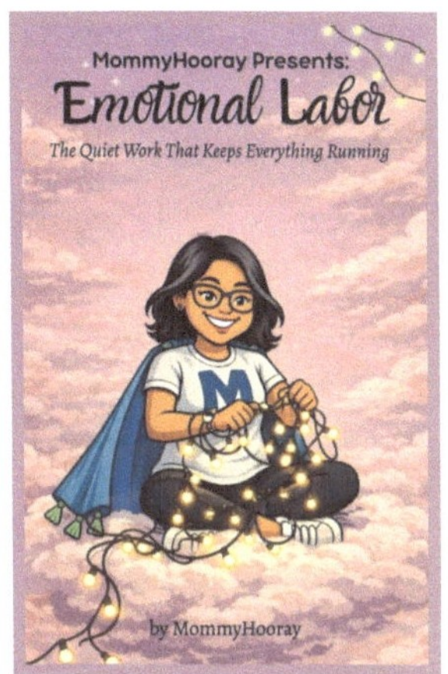

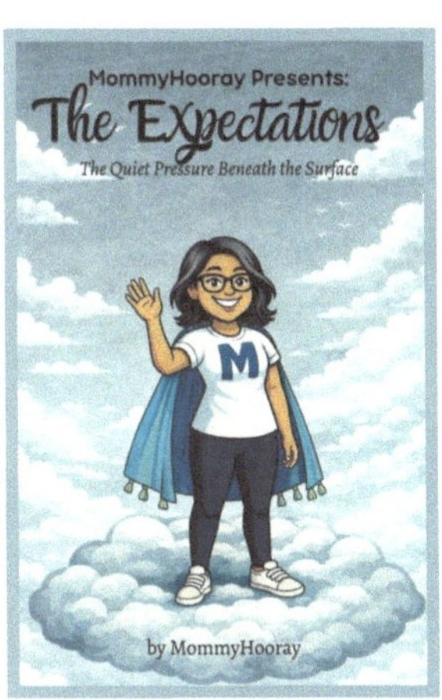

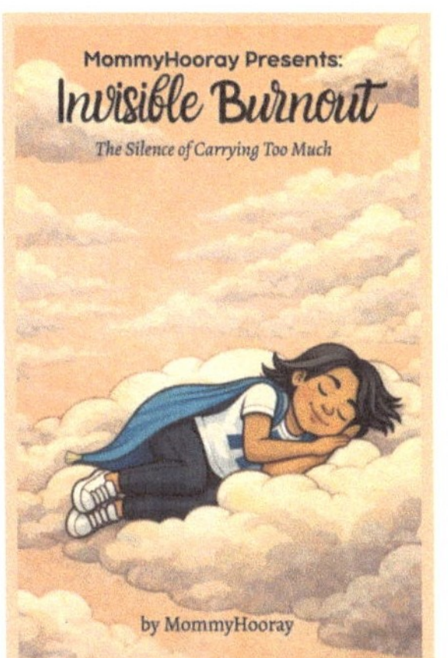

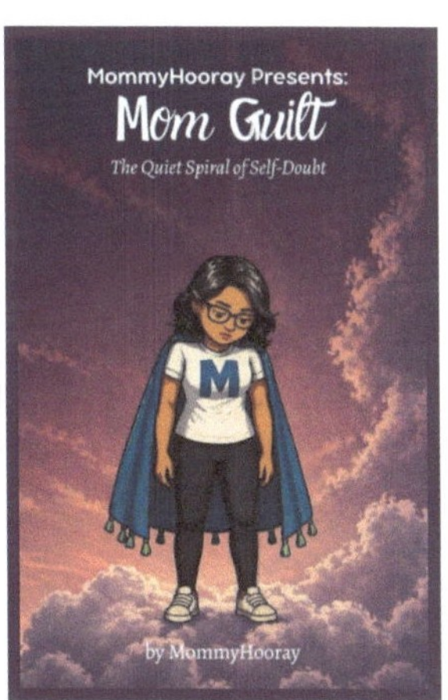

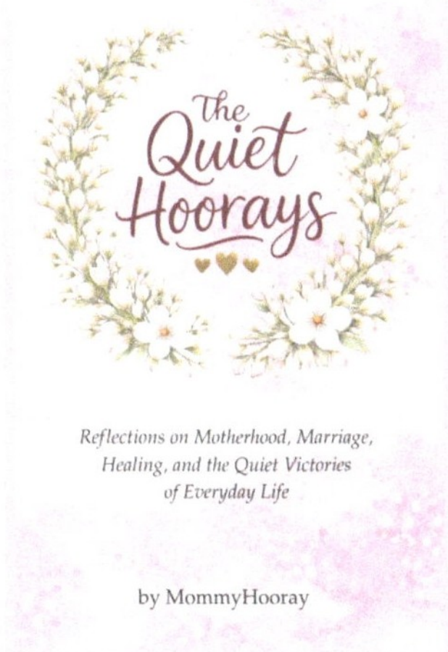

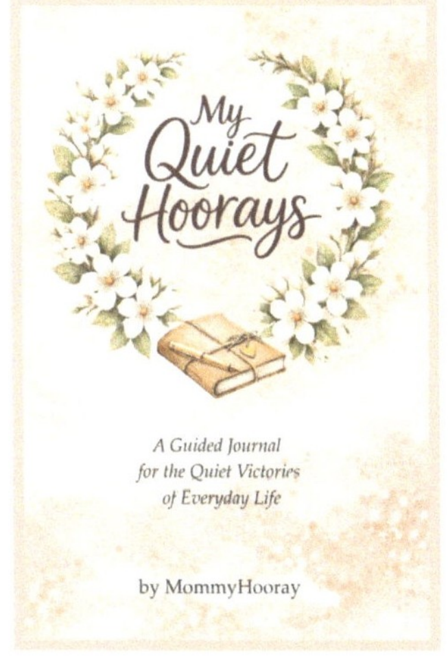

... and more!

From My Heart to Yours

Write something meaningful
for the person who will cherish this book, or for yourself.

Today's Date: ________________

May this page find you again, years from now.

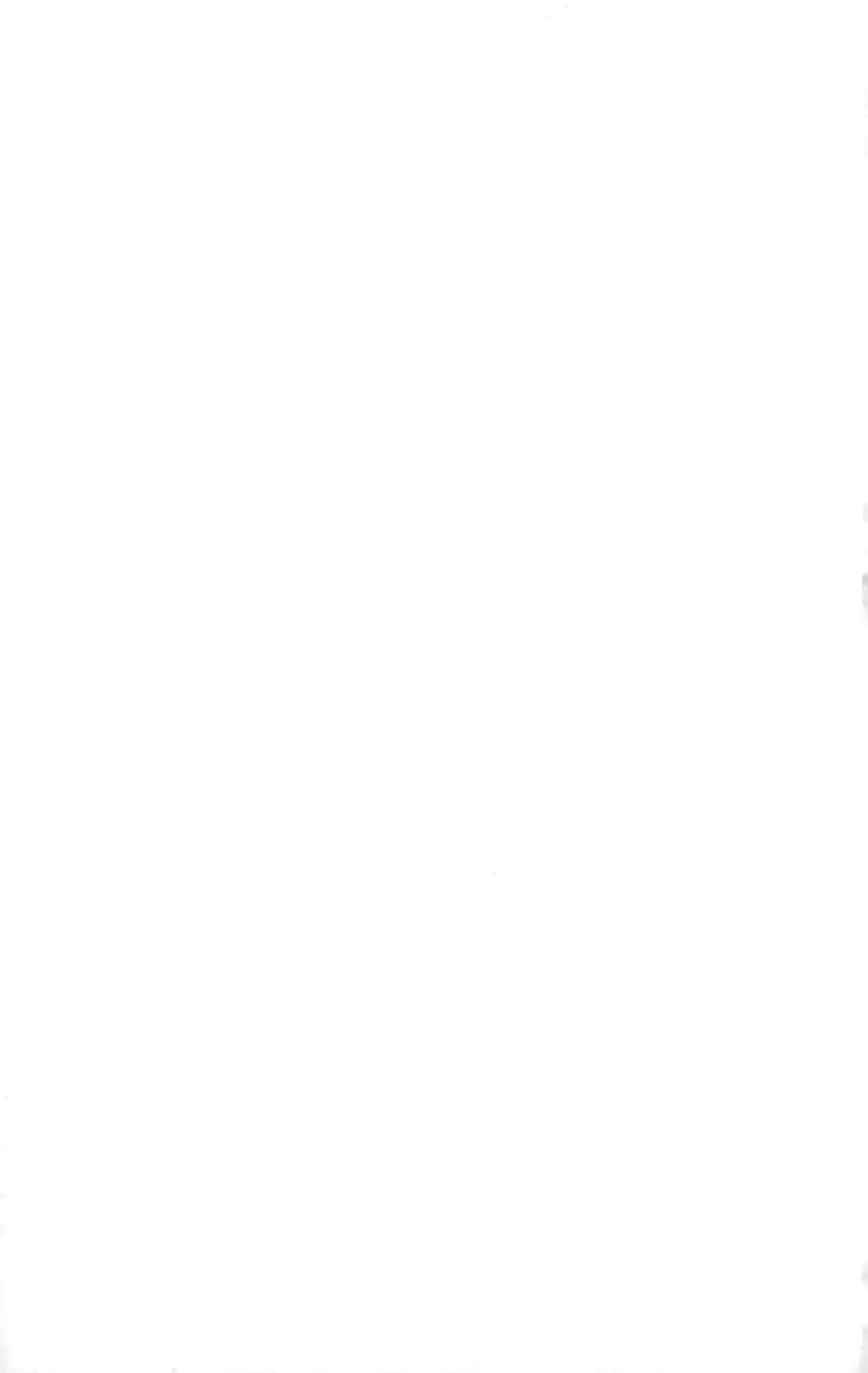

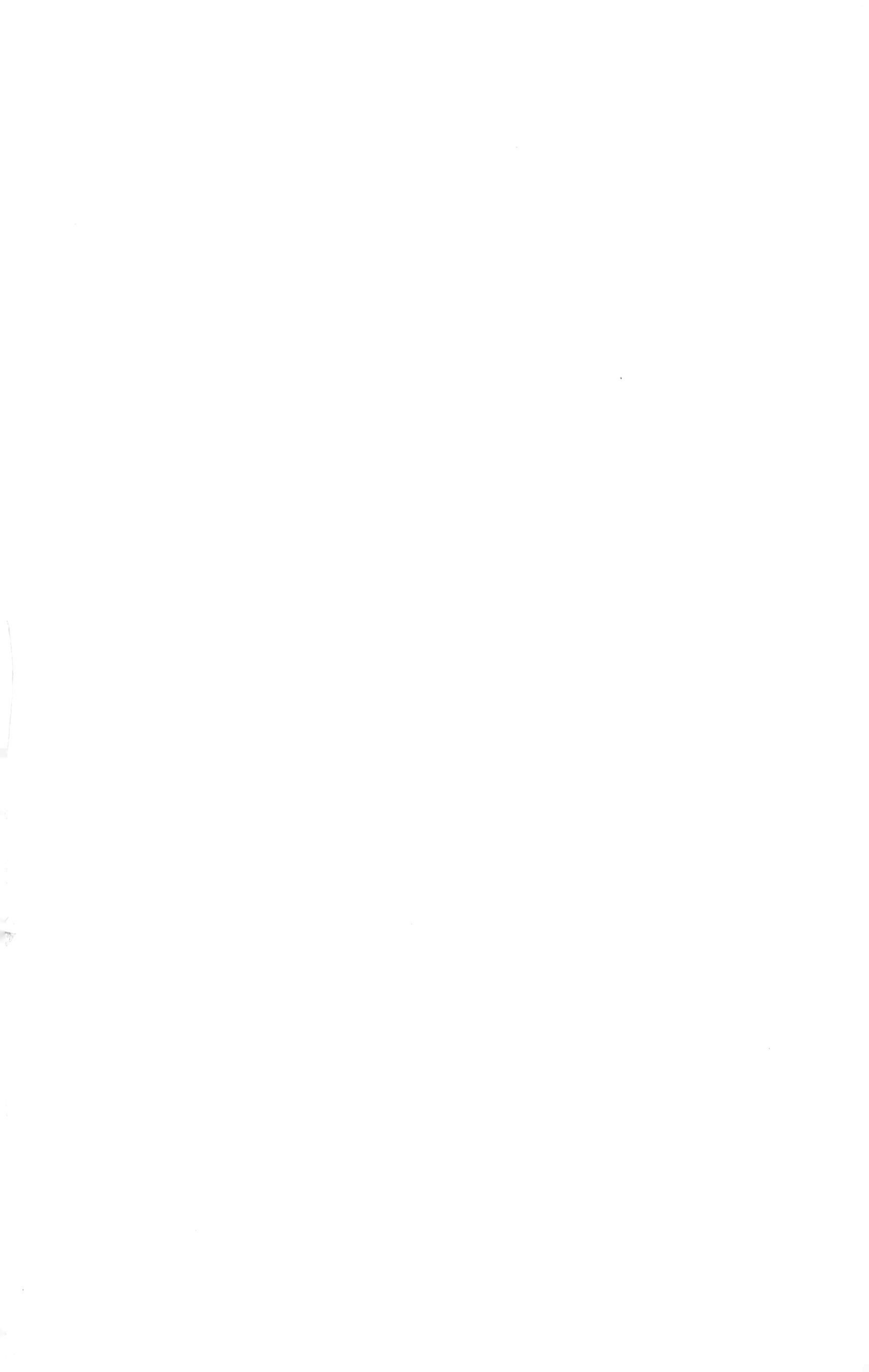

www.ingramcontent.com/pod-product-compliance
Lightning Source LLC
LaVergne TN
LVHW052259100826
845147LV00001B/89